PRIMARY
NUTRITION
Steps to Healthy Living

About the Author: Betty Wedman-St. Louis, PhD, RD, LD is a clinical nutritionist in private practice and teaches human nutrition. She believes that nutrition education can be fun and that eating habits can be changed in people of all ages.

Illustrator: Art Kirchhoff

Copyright © 2006
Milliken Publishing Company
11643 Lilburn Park Drive
St. Louis, MO 63146

www.millikenpub.com

Contents

MyPyramid: Overview

MyPyramid is the new symbol for dietary guidelines for Americans introduced in 2005. These guidelines and MyPyramid emphasize the importance of fruits and vegetables, whole grains, and healthy fats in the diet. The guidelines also recommend limiting sugar, saturated fat, and trans–fatty acids.

On April 19, 2005, the secretary of the Department of Agriculture declared, "Many Americans can dramatically improve their overall health by making modest improvements to their diets and by incorporating regular physical activity into their daily lives." MyPyramid emphasizes those guidelines by illustrating food groups and a person running up the steps of the pyramid.

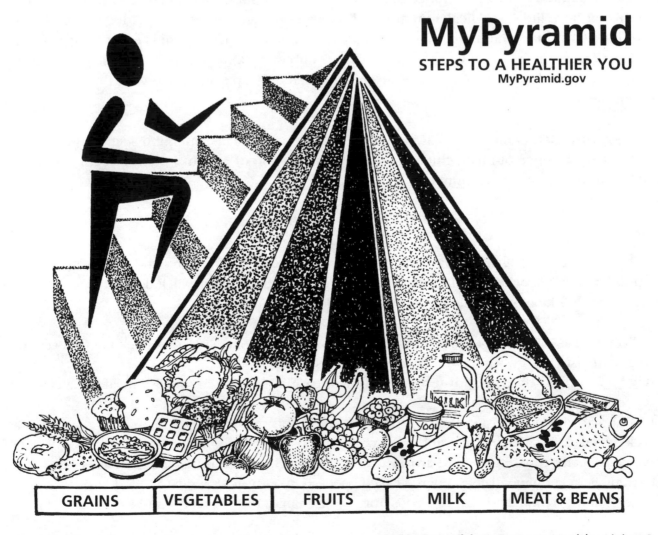

MyPyramid
STEPS TO A HEALTHIER YOU
MyPyramid.gov

| GRAINS | VEGETABLES | FRUITS | MILK | MEAT & BEANS |

Food Groups

Grains include all foods made from wheat, rice, oats, cornmeal, and barley. Examples of these foods are bread, pasta, oatmeal, breakfast cereals, tortillas, and grits. A slice of bread, 1 cup of ready-to-eat cereal, 1/2 cup of rice, pasta, or cooked cereal equals a 1-ounce serving.

Vegetables include all fresh, frozen, canned, and dried vegetables, plus vegetable juices. A cup of raw or cooked vegetables or vegetable juice, or 2 cups of raw leafy greens is considered a one cup serving.

Fruits include fresh, frozen, canned, and dried fruits. One cup of fruit, or 100% fruit juice, or 1/2 cup of dried fruit is considered a one-cup serving.

Oils include fats from many plants and fish. These fats are liquid at room temperature. Examples of healthy plant fats are canola, corn, olive, soybean, and safflower oils. Some foods are naturally high in oils such as nuts, olives, fish, and avocados. Foods that are high in fat are mayonnaise, salad dressings, and margarine.

Milk includes all fluid milk products and many foods made from milk such as yogurt and cheese. It is important to remember that foods made from milk such as cream cheese, cream, and butter that have little or no calcium are NOT a part of this group. Since most ice cream is made from high-fat cream which gives ice cream its smooth texture, ice cream is not a healthy food choice. Choose fat-free or low-fat milk foods. One cup of milk or yogurt, 1 1/2 ounces of natural cheese, or 2 ounces of processed cheese are considered 1-cup servings toward the 3-cup requirement.

Meat and Beans include meat, poultry, fish, eggs, dried beans, nuts, and seeds. Equivalent servings are 1 ounce of meat, chicken, or fish, 1 tablespoon of peanut butter, 1 egg, 1/4 cup of cooked dried beans, or 1/2 ounce of nuts or seeds.

CAUTION: Fats and Oils

To maintain caloric balance, fats and oils need to be used sparingly throughout the day. Calories from oils and fats provide a "full feeling" after eating. When good fats are included in the diet, there is usually less snacking between meals—reducing calorie consumption.

Fish such as salmon, trout, and herring are good sources of omega-3 fats. Check the FDA (Food and Drug Administration) warnings about mercury levels in fish (**www.cfsan.fda.gov/dms/admehg3.html**) before eating more than one fish meal per week.

Trans-fat labeling is required on Nutrition Facts labels as of 2006. Foods high in trans-fats such as crackers, snack foods, margarine, and fried foods should be limited in the daily diet. Sources of trans-fatty acids include hydrogenated/partially hydrogenated vegetable oils that are used to make shortening and commercially prepared baked goods. Trans-fatty acids are also found in foods from grazing animals (cattle and sheep). Foods from these animals include dairy products, beef, and lamb.

The dietary goal in fats and oils is to *reduce* saturated fats and trans-fats, while consuming proper amounts of good fats. Six teaspoons of vegetable oil per day in an 1800-calorie diet is usually adequate to meet the daily dietary need for essential fatty acids.

Physical Activity

Be active daily. An hour of moderate exercise such as walking or biking is recommended for most days. Vigorous activities like swimming are also encouraged.

Get moving!
The person running up the stairs reminds us to BE ACTIVE! Exercise everyday. Running, swimming, biking, even walking the dog are fun activities from which to choose.

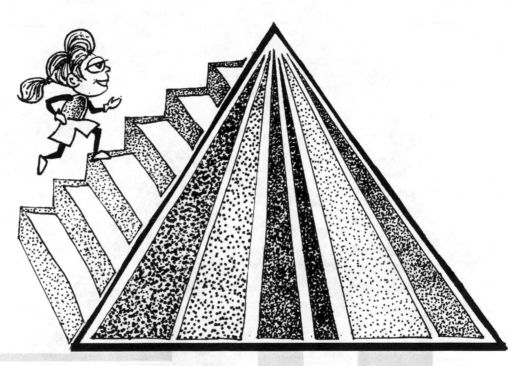

Grains 6 oz.:
Make half your grains whole. Aim for at least 3 ounces of whole grains a day.

Vegetables 2 1/2 cups:
Choose lots of colors—especially green and orange.

Fruits 1 1/2 cups:
Choose whole fruit. Make sure juices are 100% fruit.

Oils 6 tsp.:
Choose olive oil, corn oil, or canola, or oils from plants or fish.

Milk 3 cups:
Choose fat-free or low-fat calcium-rich foods.

Meat and beans 5 oz.:
Choose lean meats and other low-fat protein sources such as beans.

MyPyramid Food Match

Choosing a healthy diet requires selecting foods from all parts of the food pyramid. Place the letter of the pyramid section beside the foods listed below.

_____ 1. orange   _____ 6. hamburger   _____ 11. milk   _____ 16. oatmeal

_____ 2. cabbage   _____ 7. chicken   _____ 12. cheese   _____ 17. peanut butter

_____ 3. potato   _____ 8. hot dog   _____ 13. banana   _____ 18. broccoli

_____ 4. bread   _____ 9. beans   _____ 14. sausage   _____ 19. lettuce

_____ 5. celery   _____ 10. rice   _____ 15. cereal   _____ 20. apple

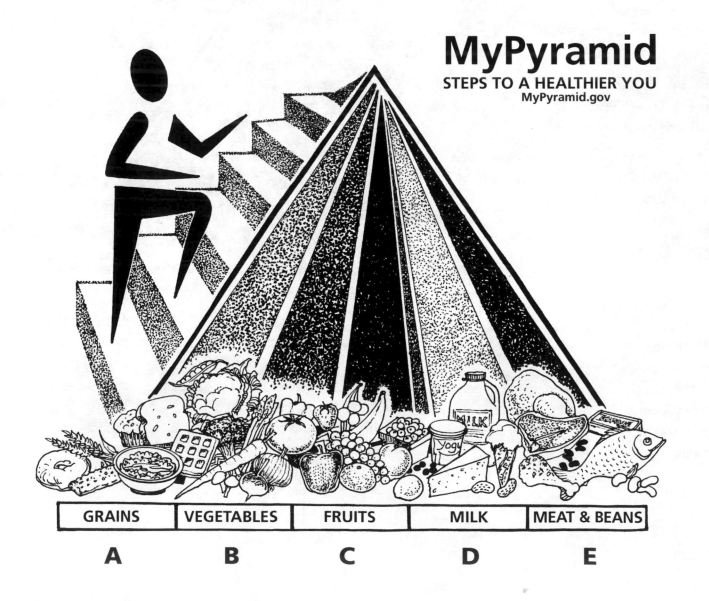

MyPyramid
STEPS TO A HEALTHIER YOU
MyPyramid.gov

GRAINS	VEGETABLES	FRUITS	MILK	MEAT & BEANS
A	B	C	D	E

Better Nutrition Through Variety

Goal: Eat foods from all food groups represented in MyPyramid.

Choosing a variety of foods from each food group increases the intake of vitamins, minerals, dietary fiber, and other essential nutrients necessary for a healthy daily diet.

Half of all **grains** eaten should be WHOLE grains. Whole grains include brown rice, bulgar, oatmeal, buckwheat, and whole-wheat crackers. Check the nutrition label for the fiber content. Whole-grain products have a higher fiber content than refined-grain foods.

Choose a wide variety of **vegetables** in different colors each day. Color-rich dark green vegetables (broccoli, spinach, kale, romaine lettuce) and orange vegetables (carrots, sweet potatoes, pumpkin, winter squash) are dense with vitamins, minerals, and fiber.

Fruits are a main source of potassium. Fruits such as bananas, cantaloupe, honeydew, prunes, oranges, apricots, peaches, and apples help reduce chronic disease, and may help maintain healthy blood pressure.

Milk, yogurt, and cheese provide calcium needed for bone health. Choose the low-fat and fat-free varieties of these foods.

Lean meats, fish, eggs, and dried beans provide a variety of important nutrients, especially protein. Low-fat cuts of meat reduce the intake of saturated fat. Fish is rich in omega-3 fatty acids, an essential fatty acid. Consider dried beans and peas as an alternative to meat.

Vegetable oils and fish oils contain polyunsaturated fatty acids. Vitamin E is also found in vegetable oils such as canola, sunflower, corn, and safflower. Nuts and avocados are other sources of healthy fats.

Ant Maze

These four ants all want the sandwich but only one is on a pathway that leads to it. Discover which ant is the lucky one? On the back of this sheet, use clues from the page to list some things you could put on the sandwich to make it healthy. Specify the best type of bread to eat.

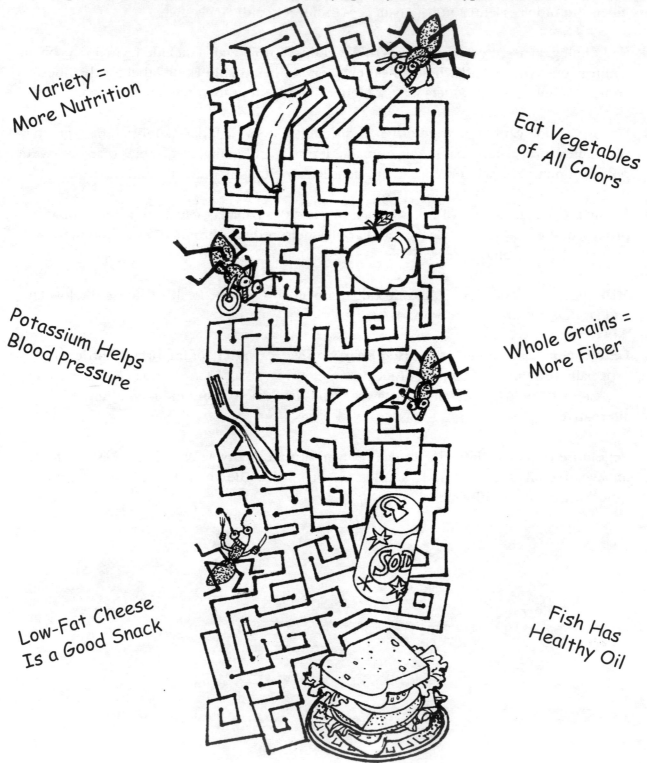

Variety = More Nutrition

Eat Vegetables of All Colors

Potassium Helps Blood Pressure

Whole Grains = More Fiber

Low-Fat Cheese Is a Good Snack

Fish Has Healthy Oil

Vegetable Word Search

Find the words listed in the WORD BANK in the puzzle below. Circle the words. Words can be horizontal, vertical, diagonal, and backwards.

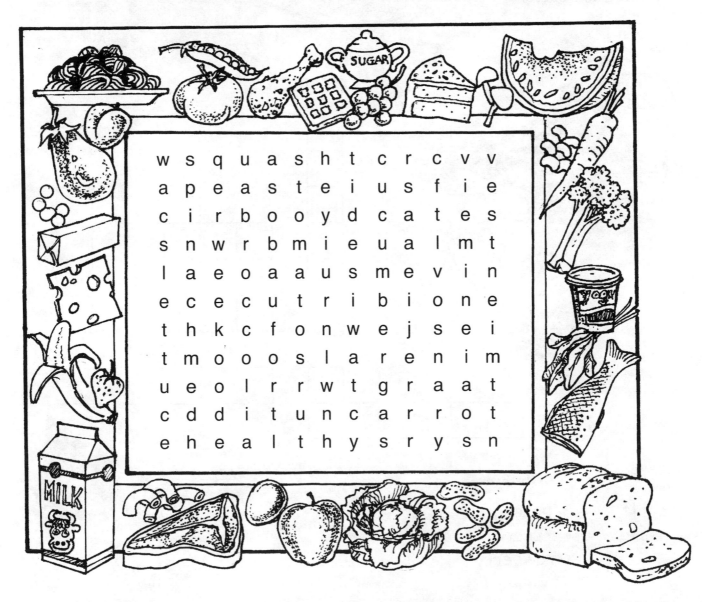

Word Bank

healthy	tomato	cucumber	squash
lettuce	corn	spinach	broccoli
carrot	peas	minerals	vitamins

```
w  s  q  u  a  s  h  t  c  r  c  v  v
a  p  e  a  s  t  e  i  u  s  f  i  e
c  i  r  b  o  o  y  d  c  a  t  e  s
s  n  w  r  b  m  i  e  u  a  l  m  t
l  a  e  o  a  a  u  s  m  e  v  i  n
e  c  e  c  u  t  r  i  b  i  o  n  e
t  h  k  c  f  o  n  w  e  j  s  e  i
t  m  o  o  o  s  l  a  r  e  n  i  m
u  e  o  l  r  r  w  t  g  r  a  a  t
c  d  d  i  t  u  n  c  a  r  r  o  t
e  h  e  a  l  t  h  y  s  r  y  s  n
```

Fruit Crossword Puzzle

Using the numbered clues and the Word Bank, solve the crossword puzzle below.

Across

4. has VITAMIN C
5. is major source of PECTIN (backwards)
6. can have seeds and increase dietary FIBER
7. may improve IMMUNE DEFENSE

Down

1. has more IRON than a raisin.
2. contains POTASSIUM
3. provides lots of FIBER

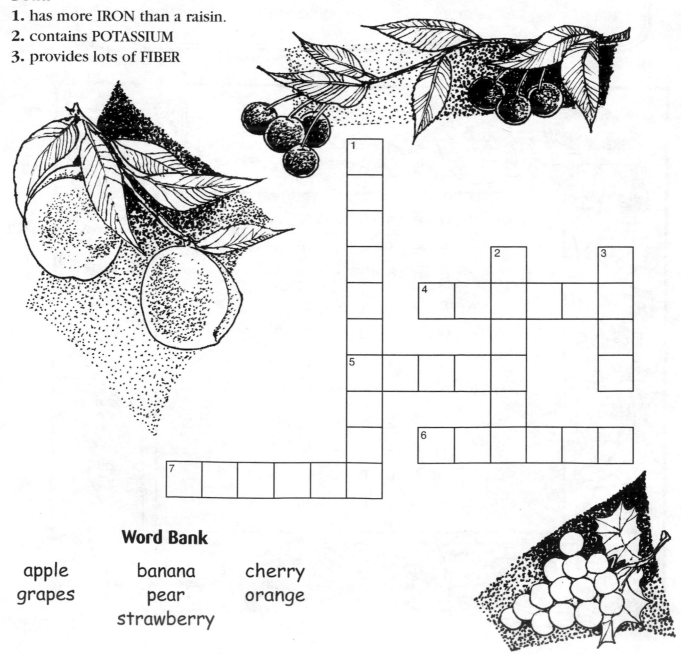

Word Bank

apple   banana   cherry
grapes   pear   orange
            strawberry

Milk Quiz

Write **T** for True or **F** for False in front of each statement about milk.

_____ 1. Whole milk is high in calcium but also high in fat.

_____ 2. Cream is high in fat and low in calcium.

_____ 3. Skim milk is a better milk choice than whole milk.

_____ 4. Low-fat yogurt is a healthy milk choice.

_____ 5. Butter is an important part of any healthy diet.

_____ 6. Butter is high in calcium.

_____ 7. High-fat cream is used to make most ice creams.

_____ 8. MyPyramid recommends a total of 2 cups of low-fat milk each day.

_____ 9. Even though it comes from milk, cream cheese does not have enough calcium to be part of the milk food group.

_____ 10. Low-fat cheese is part of the MyPyramid milk food group.

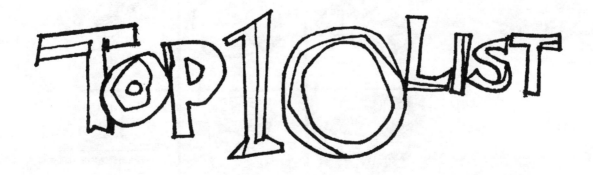

Nutrition Tic-Tac-Toe

Draw a straight line through three HIGH protein foods in the **Meat & Beans** Group.

Meat & Beans

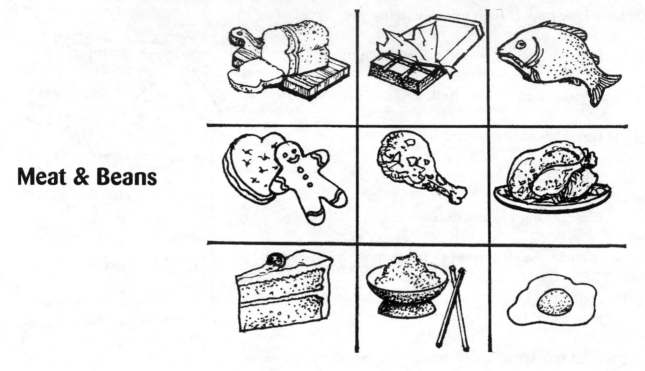

Draw a straight line through three grain foods that can be **Whole Grain** choices.

Whole Grains

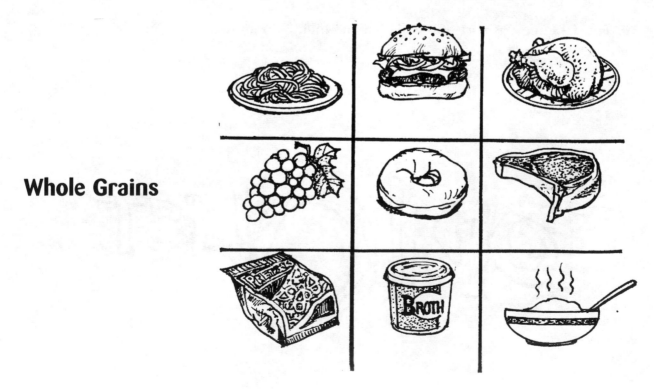

A Healthy Heart

For heart health, eat "good fats," stay away from "bad fats," and get regular exercise. Find your way through the heart maze. Circle the pictures below that show food or activities good for your heart. Put an X through the pictures that show food or activities that are bad for your heart.

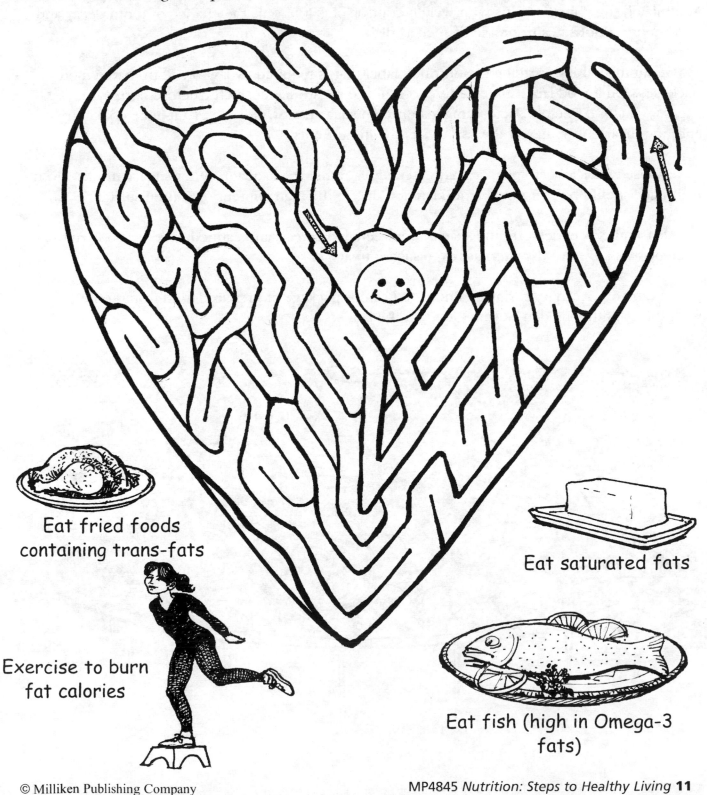

Eat fried foods containing trans-fats

Eat saturated fats

Exercise to burn fat calories

Eat fish (high in Omega-3 fats)

Don't Be Too Sweet!

Eat fewer high-sugar foods.

Choosing and preparing foods with little added sugar is an important part of a healthy diet. Minimizing sugar intake helps with weight control, plus it lessens the chance of tooth decay and other more serious health problems such as diabetes.

Get in the habit of reading the nutrition label that is required by law on all prepared food packages. On a food label, ingredients that indicate sugar include: high fructose corn syrup, sucrose, glucose, fructose, lactose, maltose, brown sugar, honey, molasses, fruit-juice concentrates, and raw sugar. Sugars have calories but are low in nutrients.

Choose water, low-fat milk, or unsweetened tea rather than soda or other sugary drinks. Even fruit juice should be consumed in moderation due to the high content of natural sugars.

Also, limit sweet desserts and snacks. Unsweetened cereals and canned fruit in 100% fruit juice or water are healthy alternatives to sugary treats.

Classroom Activity: Bring an unopened can or package of prepared food from home. Share with the class the "hidden" sugars found on the label.

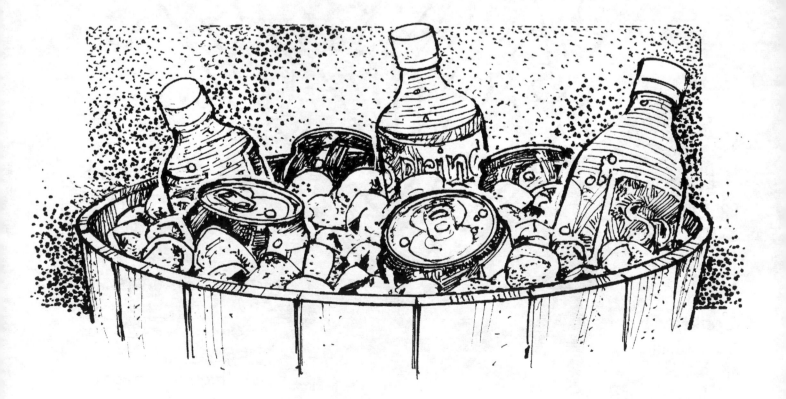

Jellybean Sugar Count

Guess the number of jellybeans in the candy jar. Write your estimate in the blank below. Using the tip printed on the label, figure out how many teaspoons of sugar and how many calories are in the jar.

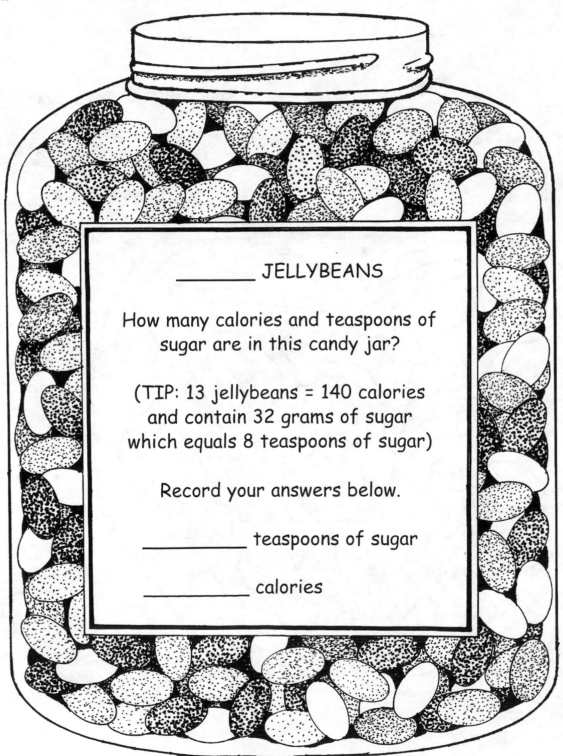

_____ JELLYBEANS

How many calories and teaspoons of sugar are in this candy jar?

(TIP: 13 jellybeans = 140 calories and contain 32 grams of sugar which equals 8 teaspoons of sugar)

Record your answers below.

_____ teaspoons of sugar

_____ calories

Ten Ways to Eat an Apple

Find your way through the apple maze. Circle the foods listed on the right that you would choose as part of a healthy diet.

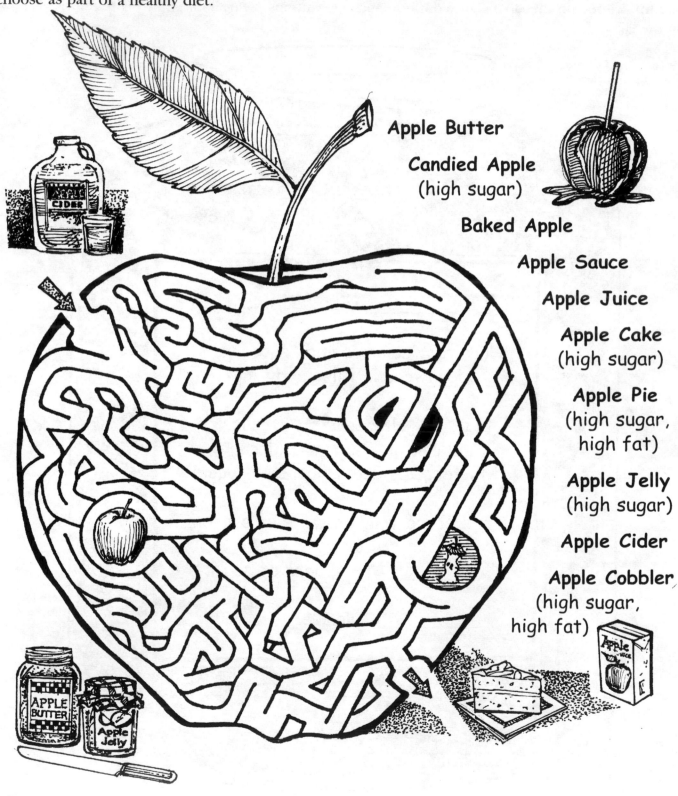

Apple Butter

Candied Apple
(high sugar)

Baked Apple

Apple Sauce

Apple Juice

Apple Cake
(high sugar)

Apple Pie
(high sugar,
high fat)

Apple Jelly
(high sugar)

Apple Cider

Apple Cobbler
(high sugar,
high fat)

Moderation

Limit intake of high-calorie, high-sugar, high-fat foods to special occasions.

Birthdays, holidays, and special events are usually celebrated with special foods. These foods are often high in sugar, fat, and calories. If you must eat these kinds of foods, remember to limit your portions.

Classroom Activity: As a class or individually, list some foods that would be tasty but healthy choices to be served for a special occasion. If you have trouble thinking of foods, look on the Internet. The National Heart, Lung, and Blood Institute Web site has a great collection of healthy dessert recipes (http://www.nhlbi.nih.gov/health/index.htm#recipes).

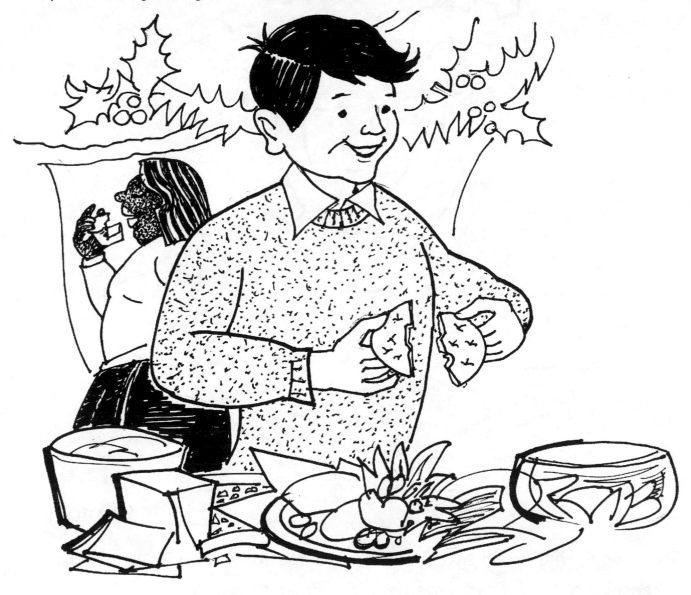

What's Wrong with This Picture?

Follow the maze through the ice-cream sundae. How many calories do you think are in the sundae? List two things this sundae contains which make it an unhealthy food choice.

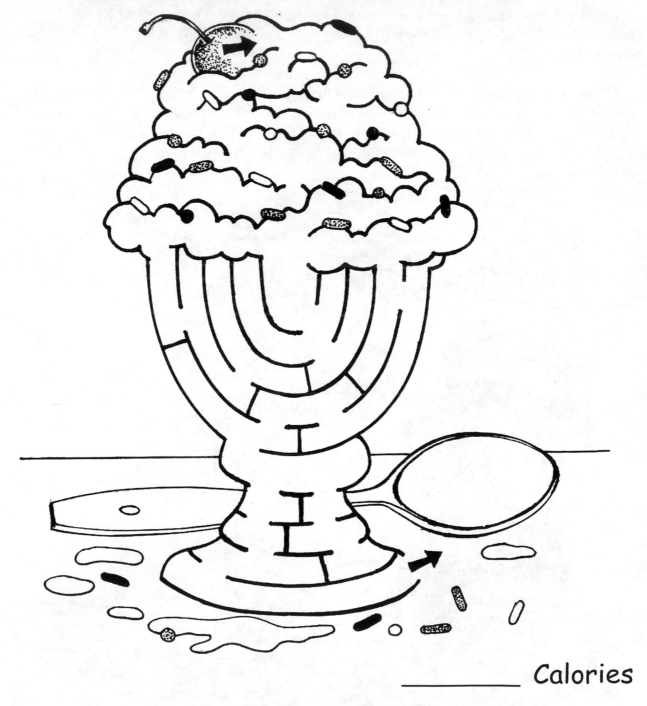

_____ Calories

Circle foods that would satisfy your sweet tooth but be a healthier choice.

Cheesecake   **Fruit Popsicle**   **Fruit Smoothie**   **Fruit Ice**

How Portions Have Changed

Look at the chart below to see how food portions have more than doubled (in many cases) over the last 20 years. It is not surprising that American waistlines have gone from **lean**

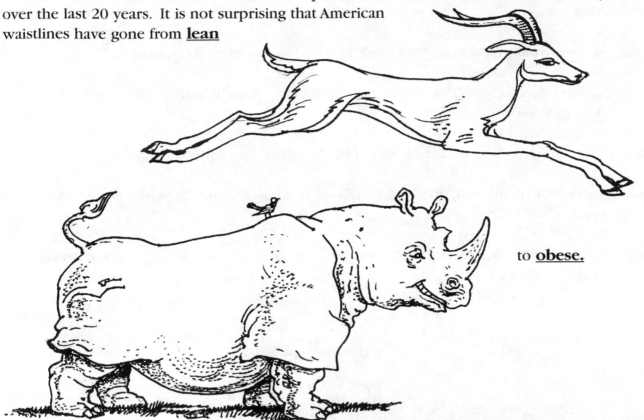

to **obese.**

Compare the portion sizes in this chart adapted from the *Portion Distortion Quiz* of the National Heart, Lung, and Blood Institute (NHLBI) Web site.

Food Item	Calories per Portion 20 Years Ago	Calories per Portion Today
Bagel	140 calories (3 in. diameter)	350 calories (6 in. diameter)
Fast-food cheeseburger	333 Calories	590 Calories
Spaghetti and meatballs	500 calories (1 cup of spaghetti with sauce and 3 small meatballs)	1,025 calories (2 cups of spaghetti and 3 large meatballs)
Bottle of soda	85 calories (6.5 oz.)	250 calories (20 oz.)
Fast-food French fries	210 calories (2.4 oz.)	610 calories (6.9 oz.)
Turkey sandwich	320 calories	820 calories (10 in. sub)

Changing Habits

Changing eating habits is not easy. Here are **5 steps to good nutrition** to encourage a gradual change in eating habits.

1. Keep healthy fruits and whole grain foods in your home. Get rid of "junk food."

2. Write down everything you eat for 2 days—be totally honest. Report to the class how this food diary changed your eating.

3. Eat smaller portions at a restaurant—don't be "force-fed" like cattle in a feedlot.

4. Learn to say, "No, thank you," to high-fat, high-sugar foods. Choose fruits, vegetables, and whole grains.

5. Reward yourself for developing good food habits by roller-blading, biking, or swimming. Avoid using food as a reward.

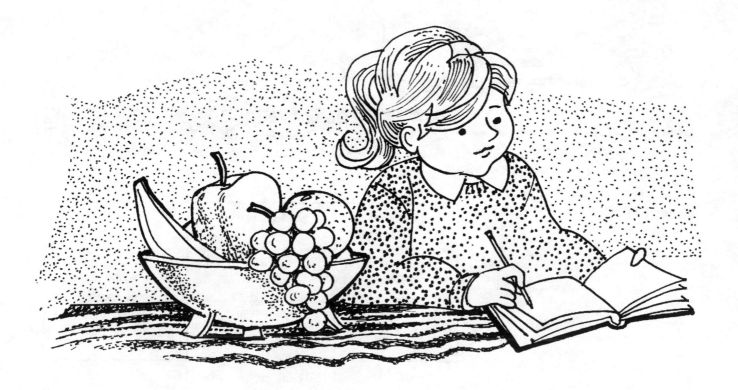

Don't Be a Couch Potato!

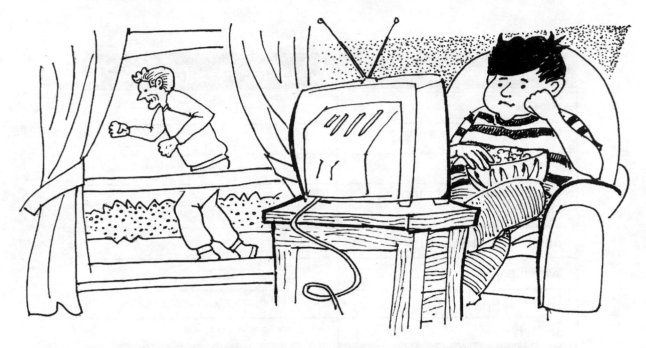

Active people can eat more than people who sit around watching television or playing video and computer games. Couch potatoes don't burn enough calories to maintain a healthy body weight.

Obesity is fast becoming a national health crisis. Excess body fat is linked with a host of life threatening diseases such as diabetes, high blood pressure, heart disease, stroke, and gall bladder disease.

Regular physical activity is a magic bullet—helping to maintain a healthy weight and reducing the risk of developing chronic health problems. At least 30 to 60 minutes a day of moderate physical activity provides many health benefits including increased bone mass during growth periods as well as decreased bone loss in old age. Children are encouraged to get 60 minutes of moderate to vigorous physical activity a day to ensure adequate bone mass development. The most important physical activities for bone health are weight-bearing exercises like jogging, walking, stair climbing, and aerobics.

The average child watches about 3 hours of television per day not including time spent watching videos and playing video and computer games. Less physical activity has resulted in more overweight children. Try to limit television and video viewing to 2 hours per day.

Classroom Activity: Using the worksheet on page 21 or another sheet of paper, keep a diet and exercise calendar for a week. After a week, share your activity log with the class. Did you come close to getting the amount of exercise needed for health? Use the chart on page 20 to determine how many calories you burned each day.

Burning Calories

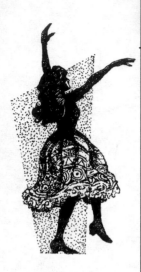

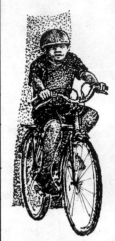

Moderate Physical Activity	cals/hr for a 154-lb. person
Hiking	367
Light gardening/yard work	331
Dancing	331
Golf (walking and carrying clubs)	331
Bicycling (<10 mph)	294
Walking (3.5 mph)	279
Weightlifting (light)	220
Stretching	184
Vigorous Physical Activity	**cals/hr for a 154 lb. person**
Running/jogging (5 mph)	588
Bicycling (>10 mph)	588
Swimming (slow freestyle laps)	514
Aerobics	478
Walking (4.5 mph)	464
Heavy yard work	441
Weightlifting (vigorous)	441
Basketball (vigorous)	441

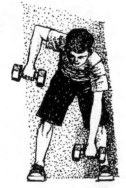

Diet & Exercise Journal

	Monday	Tuesday	Wednesday	Thursday	Friday
Breakfast					
Lunch					
Dinner					
Snack (if any)					
Physical Activity					

Physical Activity Is a Winner

Follow the maze down the mountain.

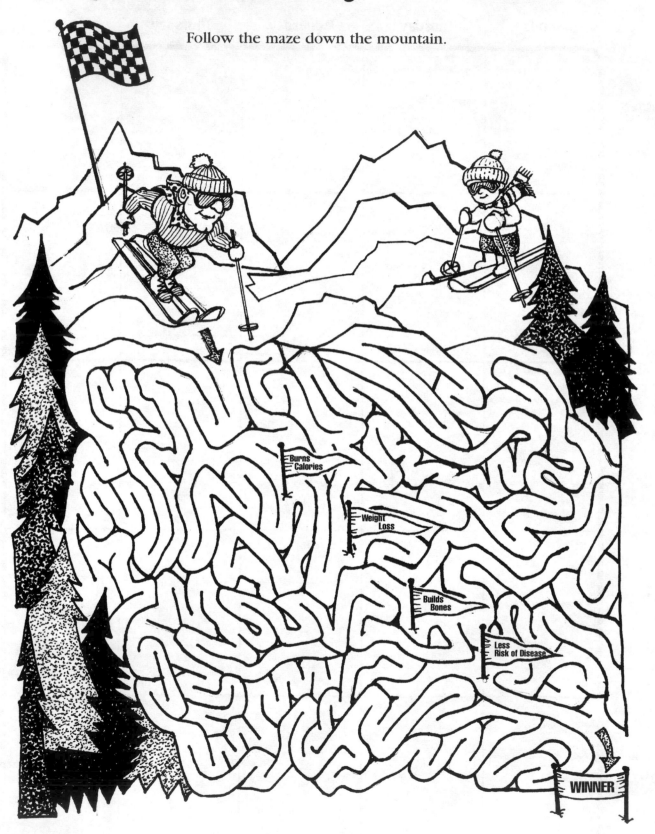

Healthy Eating

Preparing tasty new foods makes choosing healthy foods fun! Here are two recipes designed to make nutrition flavorful.

Fruit Smoothie

1 cup low-fat milk
1 cup apple juice
1 whole banana
1 cup fresh strawberries
1 cup blueberries or other seasonal fruits

Combine ingredients in blender and serve.

Spinach Salad

1 cup fresh spinach leaves
3 cups leaf lettuce or 1/4 head iceberg lettuce
1 whole diced fresh pear
1 cup sliced fresh strawberries
1/2 cup dried cranberries
1/2 cup walnut pieces
1/2 cup low-fat raspberry vinaigrette salad dressing

Combine ingredients in large bowl. Pour salad dressing over top. Toss to blend and serve.

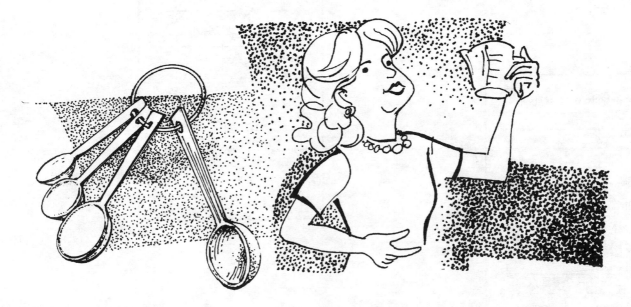

Answer Key

Page 4

1. C	6. E	11. D	16. A
2. B	7. E	12. D	17. E
3. B	8. E	13. C	18. B
4. A	9. E	14. E	19. B
5. B	10. A	15. A	20. C

Page 6

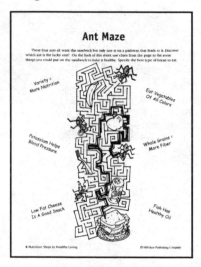

Lucky ant is right middle. Sandwich ingredients will vary. Students should choose whole-grain bread and lean meats and vegetables.

Page 7

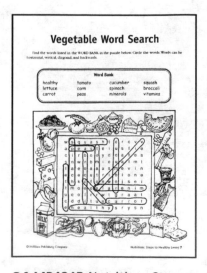

Page 8

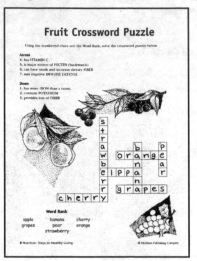

Page 9

1. T	6. F
2. T	7. T
3. T	8. F
4. T	9. T
5. F	10. T

Page 10

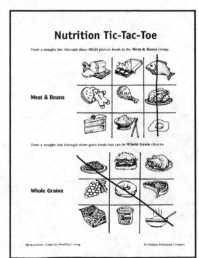

Page 11

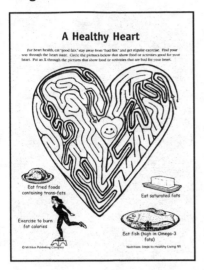

Fried chicken and butter should be crossed out. Exercise and fish should be circled.

Page 13

Answers will vary depending on jellybean estimate. If student guesses 260 beans, for example, answers would be:

260 divided by 13 = 20
20 x 140 = 2800 calories
20 x 8 = 160 teaspoons of sugar

Page 14

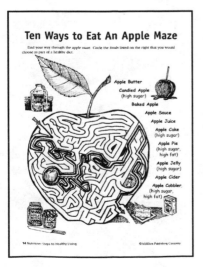

Circled apple foods are: apple butter, baked apple, apple sauce, apple juice, and apple cider.

Page 16

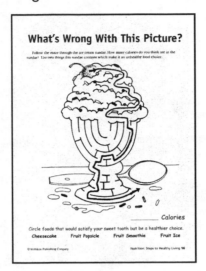

Fat and sugar (empty calories) make the ice-cream sundae a bad food choice. Healthier choices would be fruit ice, fruit smoothie, or fruit popsicle. The cheesecake has the same nutritional deficits and pitfalls as the sundae.

Page 22

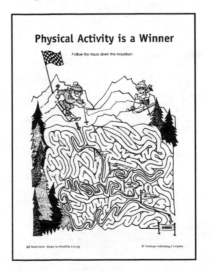

My Pyramid

MyPyramid
recommendations

Get moving!
The person running up the stairs reminds us to BE ACTIVE! Exercise every day. Running, swimming, biking, even walking the dog are fun activities to choose from.

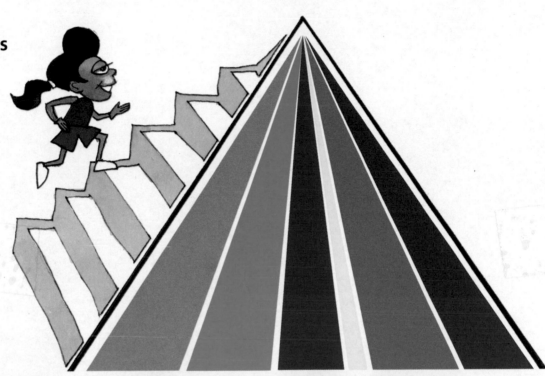

Grains
6 oz.:
Make half your grains whole. Aim for at least 3 ounces of whole grains a day.

Vegetables
2 1/2 cups:
Choose lots of colors—especially green and orange.

Fruits
1 1/2 cups:
Chose whole fruit. Juices should be 100% fruit.

Oils
6 tsp:
Choose olive oil, corn oil, or canola, or oils from plants or fish.

Milk
3 cups:
Pick fat-free or low-fat calcium-rich foods.

Meat and beans
5 oz.:
Choose low-fat meat, chicken, turkey, or fish as well as beans, nuts, and seeds.

MyPyramid Food Match

Choosing a healthy diet requires selecting foods from all parts of the food pyramid. Place the letter of the pyramid section beside the foods listed below.

_____ 1. orange	_____ 6. hamburger	_____ 11. milk	_____ 16. oatmeal
_____ 2. cabbage	_____ 7. chicken	_____ 12. cheese	_____ 17. peanut butter
_____ 3. potato	_____ 8. hot dog	_____ 13. banana	_____ 18. broccoli
_____ 4. bread	_____ 9. beans	_____ 14. sausage	_____ 19. lettuce
_____ 5. celery	_____ 10. rice	_____ 15. cereal	_____ 20. apple

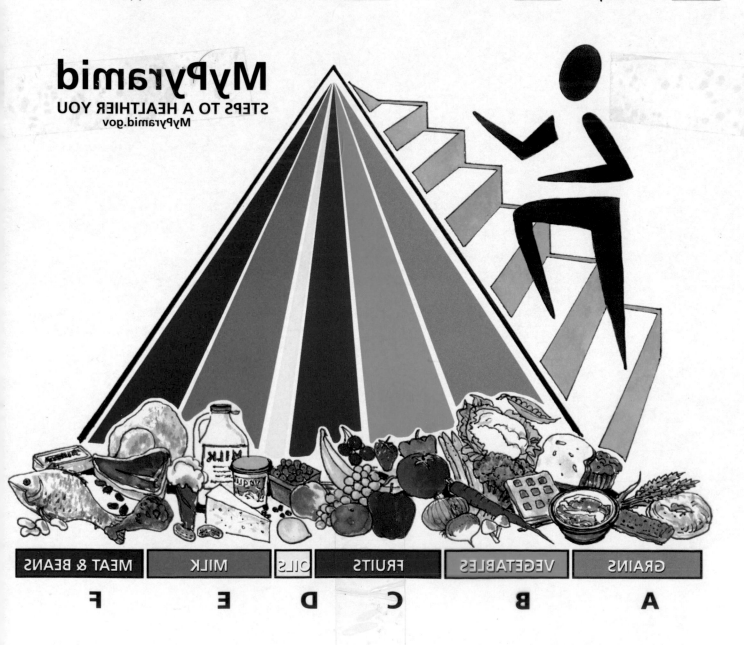

MyPyramid
STEPS TO A HEALTHIER YOU
MyPyramid.gov

A	B	C	D	E	F
GRAINS	VEGETABLES	FRUITS	OILS	MILK	MEAT & BEANS

Jellybean Sugar Count

Guess the number of jellybeans in the candy jar. Write your estimate in the blank below. Using the tip, figure out how many teaspoons of sugar and how many calories are in the jar.

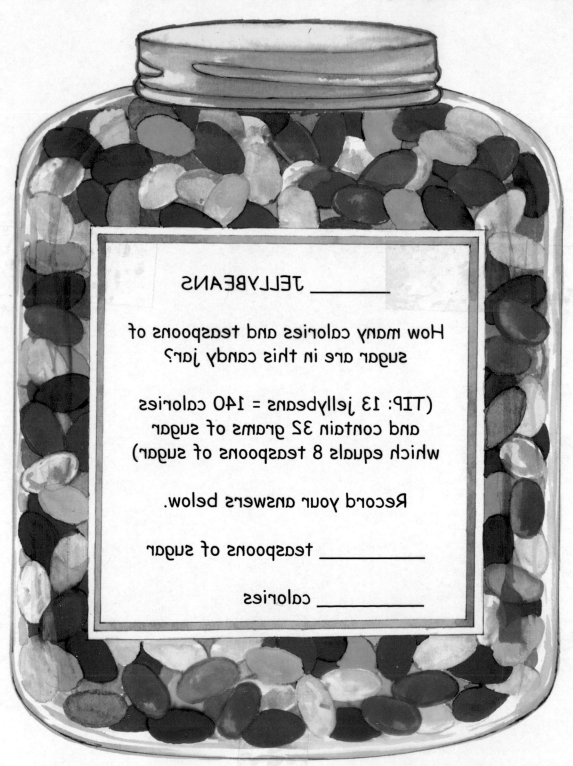

_____ JELLYBEANS

How many calories and teaspoons of sugar are in this candy jar?

(TIP: 13 jellybeans = 140 calories
and contain 32 grams of sugar
which equals 8 teaspoons of sugar)

Record your answers below.

_____ teaspoons of sugar

_____ calories

How Portions Have Changed

LEAN

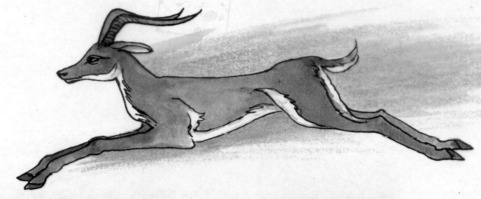

Food Item	Calories per Portion 20 Years Ago	Calories per Portion Today
Bagel	140 calories (3 in. diameter)	350 calories (6 in. diameter)
Fast-food cheeseburger	333 Calories	590 Calories
Spaghetti and meatballs	500 calories (1 cup of spaghetti with sauce and 3 small meatballs)	1,025 calories (2 cups of spaghetti and 3 large meatballs)
Bottle of soda	85 calories (6.5 oz.)	250 calories (20 oz.)
Fast-food French fries	210 calories (2.4 oz.)	610 calories (6.9 oz.)
Turkey sandwich	320 calories	820 calories (10 in. sub)

OBESE

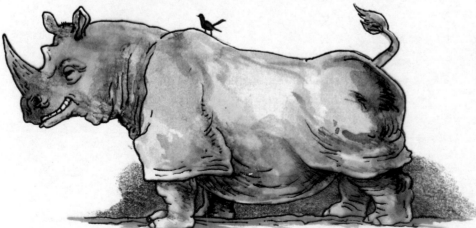

Changing Habits

Changing eating habits is not easy. Here are **5 Steps to Good Nutrition** to encourage gradual change in eating habits.

1. Keep healthy fruits and whole-grain foods in your home. Get rid of "junk food."

2. Write down everything you eat for 2 days—be totally honest. Report to the class how this food diary changed your eating.

3. Eat smaller portions at a restaurant—don't be "force-fed" like cattle in a feedlot.

4. Learn to say, "No, thank you," to high-fat, high-sugar foods. Choose fruits, vegetables, and whole grains.

5. Reward yourself for developing good habits by roller blading, biking, or swimming. Avoid using food as a reward.

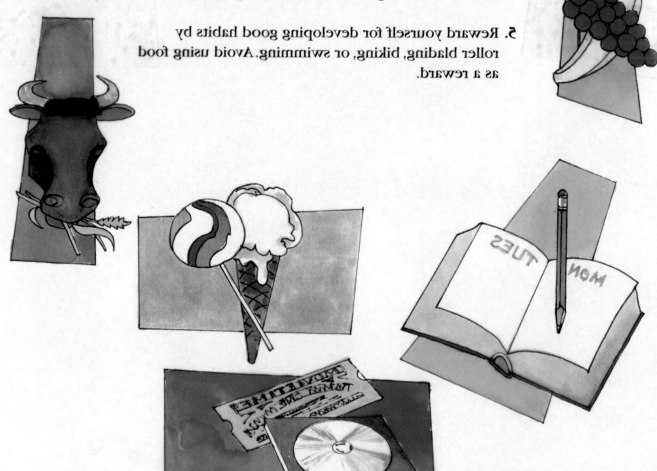

Choosing Physical Activity

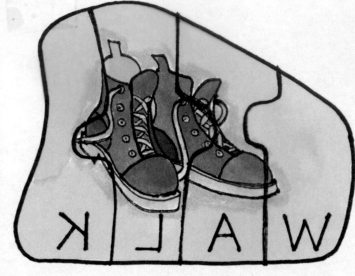

270 Calories/Hour

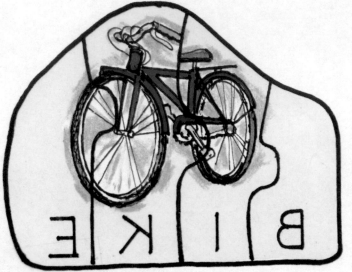

294 Calories/Hour

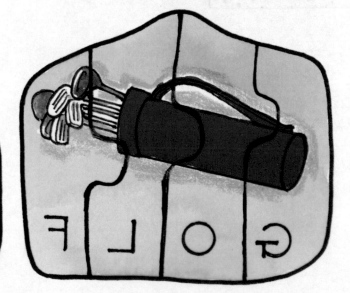

331 Calories/Hour

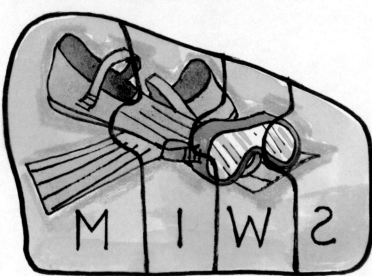

514 Calories/Hour

1 Candy Bar = 1 Hour Walking

Physical Activity

- ☐ BURNS CALORIES
- ☐ AIDS WEIGHT LOSS
- ☐ BUILDS STRONG BONES
- ☐ REDUCES TV TIME

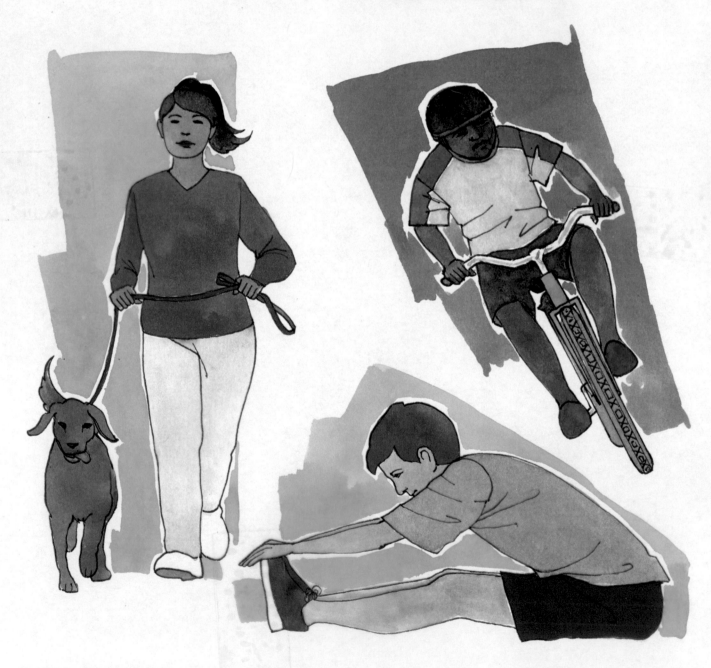

Healthy Eating

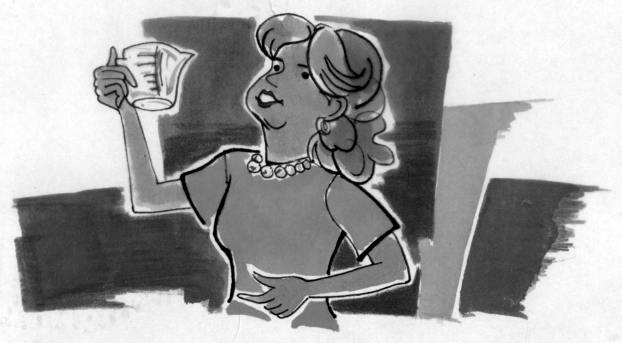

Fruit Smoothie

1 cup low-fat milk
1 cup apple juice
1 whole banana
1 cup fresh strawberries
1 cup blueberries or other seasonal fruits

Combine ingredients in blender and serve.

Spinach Salad

1 cup fresh spinach leaves
3 cups leaf lettuce or 1/4 head iceberg lettuce
1 whole diced fresh pear
1 cup sliced fresh strawberries
1/2 cup dried cranberries
1/2 cup walnut pieces
1/2 cup low-fat raspberry vinaigrette salad dressing

Combine ingredients in large bowl. Pour salad dressing over top. Toss to blend and serve.